AF824228

# What Is A Total Knee Replacement?

Melissa Cassel

INFINITY
PUBLISHING

All rights reserved. No part of this book shall be reproduced or transmitted in any form or by any means, electronic, mechanical, magnetic, photographic including photocopying, recording or by any information storage and retrieval system, without prior written permission of the publisher. No patent liability is assumed with respect to the use of the information contained herein. Although every precaution has been taken in the preparation of this book, the publisher and author assume no responsibility for errors or omissions. Neither is any liability assumed for damages resulting from the use of the information contained herein.

Copyright © 2012 by Melissa Cassel

ISBN 978-0-7414-7358-5 Paperback
ISBN 978-0-7414-7609-8 eBook

Printed in the United States of America

Published December 2012

INFINITY PUBLISHING
1094 New DeHaven Street, Suite 100
West Conshohocken, PA 19428-2713
Toll-free (877) BUY BOOK
Local Phone (610) 941-9999
Fax (610) 941-9959
Info@buybooksontheweb.com
www.buybooksontheweb.com

Do you have a sharp stabbing pain in one or both of your knees? Does it hurt every time you walk? Do you need to put a pain killer on your knee just to be able to walk?

You may need to have your knee totally replaced. It is important that you get your knees x-rayed to find out what the problem is. Many baby-boomers are needing to have their knees replaced. People are more active in this age group. They want to do what they did when they were younger. One of the reasons for weak knees, is being overweight, or genetics can contribute.

The pain is not going to go away unless you take care of the problem. I know it happened to me. You need to set up your living place before you go to the hospital. The carpet on the stairs should not be loose. Walk through the house and make sure that all of the throw rugs are out of the way.

You need to keep the items that are used often in the kitchen at waist level. If you do not have little children, use the front burners on the stove. The pots and pans slide them along the counter.

The furniture should be strong enough to lean on. You should put a pillow in the recliner, so that you can get out of your favorite chair easier. Before surgery you should plan to not have clutter. You cannot climb onto footstools when you are recovering from your operation. Check with your doctor before surgery of what you can and cannot do after the operation. You might want to remove any coffee tables.

The supplies that you should have before surgery are an apron with several pockets, a steady stool when you are doing countertop chores, a reacher, or a long handle dustpan. On your walker you can put a walker tray on it, or a walker bag or basket. This can be used to carry plates, silverware and food is in sealed containers.

If you have a pet you might want to get dry food before surgery. This will help you not to bend down so much. You should move your clothing where you can get to it easily. I suggest that you use the walker basket for small laundry items. The reacher can aid you in getting the clothes from the back of the dryer or the bottom of the washer.

You should receive help with heavy cleaning, such as vacuuming or scrubbing the bathtub when you are recovering. Always avoid problems. You should have a long telephone extension, that is near your chair, or an easy to reach light switch.

When using the bathroom have a toilet raiser. You will also need a handrail to get up. You should not bend or force your knee past what the doctor has told you until he or she gives you permission. Have a reacher by the toilet at all times.

When giving yourself a bath use a tall bath bench or chair. Make sure that a non-skid surface is in an out of the bathtub. The supplies that you will need, bathbrush, shampoo, soap, towels, and your clothing. They should be easy to get to. Have a bucket to keep all of the bath items together. You can use soap on a rope, so that you do not have to bend down. There is also no rinse shampoo. You should use an extended shower hose that has an on/ off button in the tub or shower.

Always be sure and follow safety with your knee. You should not take your walker or crutches into the shower. You should swing your legs over the bathtub. Always wear shoes. You will need to put towels on the floor of the bathroom. You should dry yourself off before getting out of the shower.

When dressing you will need help. A sock aid will help you with putting on socks. I found it easy for me to sit on my bed and dress myself. I always had a reacher with me to pull up my socks and slacks. I found slip on shoes were the easiest to put on my feet.

Exercise is very important to your recovery. You will need to do two complete sets of exercises, everyday including weekends, in order to get full usage of your leg and knee. You can use your bed for many exercises. You may also use chairs and stairs.

Shortly after the operation, you will start to walk in the hospital room and work on every day activities. This will help you with your recovery. This is the best way to help you regain your ability to use your knee. The doctor will tell you how much weight you can put on the leg. You will start with your walker or crutches. You will need to walk as smooth as you can.

You will need a handrail at first to go up and down the stairs. You will work on this more than likely in physical therapy. Stair climbing will help you with strength and endurance. I found this saying to be helpful, "up with the good and down with the bad." You should always use a handrail for balance.

These are the exercises that you will probably do in physical therapy, ankle pumps and circles, thigh squeezes, heel slides, leg slides, lying kicks, straight leg raises, knee bending, prolonged knee stretch, sitting kicks, knee straightening stretch, knee straight leg dangling, swinging, buttocks squeezes, hamstring sets, straight leg raises, knee straightening exercises, bed-supported knee bends, sitting supported knee bends, standing knee bends, assisted knee bends, knee exercises with resistance and exercycling. There are many machines that are used in the physical therapy department. I found it important to go to physical therapy. The reason is that there are some exercises that you cannot do at home without the machines. Also the therapist will make sure that you are doing the exercise correctly.

There are exercises that I found that are very important to do. Get a chair, then place a pillow on the seat of the chair place your affected knee on the pillow and lean into the chair, pushing forward. You hold this for 1:00 minute each time. Do this twice a day. This will help to loosen the scar tissue.

There is another exercise that is important. You will need a 5 pound bag of flour or sugar, put in a double plastic bag. You then have your leg stretched out on a sturdy chair. You then take both of your hands and press down hard on the bag of sugar or flour and press down 5 times holding for 1:00 minute each time. Do this twice a day. This helps with the swelling of the knee.

There is another exercise that was important. Take a towel wrap it around your affected ankle. Pull your foot towards you and hold for 5 seconds. You should do this 5 times. You should do this twice a day. Always be sure and get your doctors permission before doing any exercise.

The reason why exercise is important, is that it speeds up recovery, joints heel faster, you feel better quicker. Every person recovers at his or her own rate.

Eating properly is important before and after surgery. The foods that are high in phosphorus and vitamin d are yogurt, broccoli, cheese, puddings and Carnation Instant Breakfast. If you cannot drink milk talk to your doctor about this. These foods are high in protein, milk and dairy products, beef, turkey, eggs, breads and cereal, nuts, pork, chicken, game meats, fish, beans and peanut butter.

These foods are high in vitamin a, apricots, carrots, mangoes, pumpkin, potatoes, tomato juice, almonds, bananas, cashews, whole wheat bread and spinach.

The foods that are high in vitamin c, are broccoli, Brussels sprouts, cantaloupe, cabbage, cauliflower, collard greens, grapefruit juice, grapefruit, kale, kiwi, lemons, mangos, orange juice, oranges, peppers,(sweet, red and green), strawberries and potato skins.

There are many ways to increase your protein intake:

**CIB Shake**

- 1 envelope Carnation Instant Breakfast
- 1 c of whole milk
- 1/4 c non fat dry milk powder
- 3 scoops of ice cream
- Add extracts, fruit or flavored syrup for variety
- Calories 353 Protein 16.5 g

**CIB Shake – Low Calorie Option**

- 1 envelope sugar free Carnation Instant Breakfast
- 1 c of skim milk
- 1/4 c non fat dry milk powder
- 3 scoops low fat ice cream
- Add extracts or fruit for variety
- Calories 239 Protein 16.4 g

**Fruit Salad Smoothie**

- 1c of fruit juice
- 1c of tofu or yogurt
- 2 kiwi peel and cut into chunks
- 1/2 c fresh pineapple
- 1 large banana
- 1 c of strawberries
- 2Tbsp honey

Place all ingredients into a blender, puree until smooth. Serve garnished with additional whole fruit. Note: Other fruit maybe used, such as melons, raspberries, papayas or mangoes. Yields 4 1 c servings. Calories 180 per serving.

## Things You Need To Know

- Take a good pair of shoes with you.
- You will need to take loose fitting clothes.
- You can generally wear your own clothes the day after surgery.
- Take your own personal items, except rings and watch.
- Let family members help you.
- Limit visitors to conserve energy.
- Anyone that is sick should not see you.
- Make sure someone can take you and pick you up from the hospital.
- If you are a shorter person your knee will probably swell. This is because your body is more compact. The swelling of your knee will more than likely go down in two months.

# Things You Need To Know

- You will be receiving a plastic card in the mail with the date of the implant and the surgeon's name. You will need to keep this in your wallet for future reference.
- You will need to tell your dentist or any other doctor about your total knee replacement. You will need to take antibiotics before going to the dentist. The length of time depends on the surgeon that did your operation.
- The hospital stay will probably be 2 to 6 days.
- The total knee replacement cannot make you younger.
- The rehabilitation exercises are for the knee to recover.
- It can be uncomfortable doing the exercises.
- You will regain the function that you are going to get in more than likely six months to a year.

# Things You Need To Know

- You will more than likely need two months of physical therapy.
- If you do not do the exercises you will be pain free and the function of your knee will more than likely not improve.
- If you do not do the therapy immediately you cannot catch up, as the knee will stiffen.
- The reason to have a total knee replacement is to lower the pain by arthritis or injury to the knee joint.
- The implant is size specific and not gender specific.
- There is not a cast, just a dressing covering where the cut was made.
- When you work a desk job you may be able to return in a few weeks. If your job requires heavy lifting, it is possible to be out for several months.
- A total knee replacement replaces all of the joint.
- You should pick your doctor and hospital carefully.
- You will need to tell your doctor of any allergies to drugs. Also be sure and tell the anesthesiologist if you are sensitive to anesthesia.

## Things You Need To Know

- The exercises focus on full body strength.
- The therapist will manually manipulate to help restore movement.
- You will become tired easily.
- It is possible that it will take up to a year to build your endurance back.
- It is important to force yourself each day to do a little more.
- It will more than likely take many months for a full recovery. Remember it is worth the effort.
- If your doctor has told you that you need a knee replacement you should not delay.
- Delaying surgery will possibly lower the quality of life before and two years after surgery.
- The way the knee replacement works depends on age, weight and your activity level.
- Your surgeon will order medical tests before the operation to make sure you are healthy.

## Things You Need To Know

- To be prepared for surgery you may need to lose weight and quite smoking.
- Tell your surgeon if you are taking aspirin or other medications.
- You will more than likely start your rehabilitation within 24 hours.
- Each day you will probably increase your daily activities.
- It is normal to run a low grade fever for a few days after the surgery.
- You should check with your doctor before doing high impact activities.
- Six to twelve weeks after surgery there are some exercises that may be added, toe and heel raiser, partial knee bends and step ups.
- The ability to drive depends on how you are recovering. This is generally 4 to 6 weeks later. Right knee replacements sometimes take longer to recover.

## Things You Need To Know

- There are patients that decide to recover at a rehabilitation center. The decision depends on if you have family and friends that will help you during your recovery period.
- You should talk with your family several weeks before surgery and how they can help you.
- Osteoarthritis, rheumatoid arthritis and trauma related arthritis are the most common reasons for joint damage.
- Osteoarthritis results in the smooth joint surfaces to erode. This causes, bone on bone contact, pain, stiffness and swelling. Bone spurs can grow on edges of the joint.
- You should turn your entire body to avoid stress on your knee.
- Do not push yourself to hard.
- You will be given a physical exam to measure your range of motion of your hips, knees and check on your muscle strength.
- The doctor will watch how you walk, sit, bend and move.
- X-Rays will be taken of your knee joint.
- If you have any X-Rays of your knee you should take them to the doctor's appointment.

# Things You Need To Know

- The physical therapist will teach you the safest ways for getting in and out of bed, chair and going up and down the stairs.
- The therapist will want to know about your living environment.
- You may be using a passive motion machine a (CPM), this gently bends and straightens your knee automatically.
- It is time to get your knee X-Rayed when pain medication will not help.
- Only an orthopedic surgeon can tell you whether an implant is ok for you.
- Knee pain can limit your activities.
- The surfaces of the knee roll and glide against each other as the knee bends.
- If you have osteoarthritis everyday activities can be painful if not impossible. Things like walking, driving and standing may cause you extreme pain.
- Ask your doctor before doing cross country skiing, table tennis, bowling and rowing, after surgery.
- You should elevate your knee in bed.
- I found sleeping in a recliner is easier than trying to sleep in bed, especially for the first month. It also makes it easier to get to the bathroom at night.
- You will probably be taking a blood thinner until your scheduled appointment with the doctor to remove the sutures.

## Things You Need To Know

- Surgery is recommended when you cannot walk any distance, medications do not help and your sleep is interrupted.

- There are potential risks.

- Your surgeon may ask you to donate blood before the operation in case you need a transfusion for surgery.

- There are medications that can help you manage pain during physical therapy.

- When you are at the hospital your daily activities will include, sitting on the side of the bed, walking a few steps with a cane, crutches or walker, sitting in a chair and transferring yourself to a bedside commode.

- The third day and until you leave, bend your knee to a 90 degree angle, or show improvement in bending the knee, straighten the knee, walk with little effort with a cane, crutches or walker, move to a chair or commode without help and dress yourself, climb possibly seven steps.

- At six weeks you will probably no longer need to use a walker or crutches.

# Things You Need To Know

- At twelve weeks you can enjoy a variety of low impact activities such as swimming, walking, golfing and bicycling.
- Your doctor will tell you when you can walk without a cane.
- If you have no problems you will be able to walk on your own.
- You will be told when you can increase your household routine, such as cooking, cleaning and your laundry.
- You will be able to take a shower after your incision has healed.
- In many cases you will start with smaller height steps and move to standard height steps.
- After three months your physical therapist may have you do more strengthening and stretching exercises.
- A sock aid helps you put on socks without bending.
- You should not wax hard wood floors where you live.

# Things You Need To Know

- Knee replacement surgery was first done in 1968.
- Total knee replacements are successful.
- There are more than 600,000 knee replacements that are performed each year in the United States.
- It is best to have the surgery in the spring or summer.
- You need healthy knees to perform daily activities.
- There is no absolute age or weight restrictions for total knee replacements.
- Most people range in age from 50 to 80.
- Surgery is based on a patient's pain and disability not their age.
- Any infection in your body can spread to your joint replacement.

# Things You Need To Know

- Scarring of the knee can occasionally happen.
- There is a small number of patients that have a continued knee pain after the replacement. This does not happen very often.
- Injury to the nerve or blood vessels around the knee can occur during surgery. This is rare.
- The operation generally takes between 1 and 2 hours.
- You will be in the recovery room for several hours.
- You should be able to resume daily living activities in 3 to 6 weeks.
- For several weeks after surgery you may have pain at night.
- Kneeling after surgery is sometimes uncomfortable but it is not harmful.
- Your new knee may activate metal detectors that is required for security in airports and other buildings. Tell them about your knee replacement.

## Things You Need To Know

- With modification the knee replacement can last many years.
- Serious problems, such as knee joint infection occurs in fewer than 2% of patients.
- For several weeks after surgery you may have pain at night.
- Women who are over 50 are more likely to develop osteoarthritis of the knee than men.
- The ability of cartilage to heal itself decreases as people age.
- Osteoarthritis affects 40 million Americans.
- Osteoarthritis can cause financial stress because many patients with the condition can no longer work.
- There are times when both knees need to be replaced at the same time.

## Things You Need To Know

- Osteoarthritis of the knee is one of the five main causes of disability among senior citizens.
- The risk is great for disability from osteoarthritis.
- Osteoarthritis happens when the knee has been injured or infected.
- There are jobs that put you at a higher risk for knee problems, assembly line worker, dock worker, miner and carpet floor layer.
- There are certain illnesses that can increase your chances for knee problems, gout and metabolic problems.
- Injuries to the knee such as sport injuries can lead to problems of the knee.
- It is possible to feel pain by sitting or lying down if you are having knee problems.

# Things You Need To Know

- The knee is the largest joint in the body.
- Osteoarthritis can result in bone rubbing on bone.
- Bone spurs are common in osteoarthritis.
- Surgery is suggested when there is pain or stiffness, inflammation, bowing in or out of your knee, other treatments do not work.
- There are more than 90%of people who have total knee replacement that have a significant improvement.
- There are different types of knee implants.
- It is common to have shallow breathing after surgery. The nurse will have you take deep breaths.

## Things You Need To Know

- A balanced diet is important before and after surgery.
- There can be some loss of appetite several weeks after surgery.
- Iron is important in your diet to help your wound heal and to give you muscle strength.
- After surgery continue to be in regular light exercise programs.
- You should have a temporary living space on the ground floor. The reason is that walking up and down stairs will be difficult during your early recovery.
- The thigh muscles give the knee stability.

## Things You Need To Know

- Most people are admitted to the hospital on the same day as the surgery.
- You should have steady handrails on your stairways.
- You should have safety bars or handrails in your shower or bath.
- You should move your foot and ankle after surgery for increased blood flow in your leg muscles and prevent swelling and blood clots.

# Bibliography of Sources

The American Academy of Orthopedic Surgeons 6300 N. River Road Rosemont, IL 60018 Telephone Number: 1-847-823-7186

Levine, Beth : Everything You Need To Know About New Knees AARP: March 2011 : Pages 12-16

St. Jon's Center for Orthopedic Care (Now Called Mercy) Joplin, Missouri Telephone Number : 1-417-625-2369

Made in the USA
Monee, IL
04 November 2026

67377643R00015